A LITTLE BOOK OF NURSES' RULES

S0-ASM-412

A LITTLE BOOK OF NURSES' RULES

ROSALIE HAMMERSCHMIDT, R.N.
Manager of Clinical Resource Utilization
Saint Thomas Hospital, Nashville, Tennessee

CLIFTON K. MEADOR, M.D.
Director of Medical Affairs, Saint Thomas Hospital
Clinical Professor of Medicine, Vanderbilt University
　School of Medicine, Nashville, Tennessee

Philadelphia
HANLEY & BELFUS, INC.

Published by HANLEY & BELFUS, INC., 210 S. 13th Street,
Philadelphia, PA 19107. (215) 546-7293; 800-962-1892.

North American and worldwide sales and distribution:
Mosby, 11830 Westline Industrial Drive, St. Louis, MO 63146
In Canada: Times Mirror Professional Publishing, Ltd., 130 Flaska Drive,
Markham, Ontario, Canada L6G 1B8

Designed by Adrianne Onderdonk Dudden

A LITTLE BOOK OF NURSES' RULES   ISBN 1-56053-065-0
© 1993 by Rosalie Hammerschmidt, R.N.
   and Clifton K. Meador, M.D.

All rights reserved. No part of this book may be reproduced, reused, republished, or
transmitted in any form or by any means without written permission of the publisher.
Library of Congress catalog card number 92-75322

Last digit is the print number: 9 8 7 6 5 4 3 2 1

Other Books of Interest from HANLEY & BELFUS, INC.

THE BEST OF NURSING HUMOR, by Colleen Kenefick and Amy Young, 1993, $25.00

THE BEST OF MEDICAL HUMOR, by Howard J. Bennett, MD, 1991, $25.00

A LITTLE BOOK OF DOCTORS' RULES, by Clifton K. Meador, MD, 1993, $8.95

DICTIONARY OF MEDICAL ACRONYMS & ABBREVIATIONS, 2nd ed., by Stanley Jablonski, 1992, $15.95

THE SECRETS SERIES® Charles M. Abernathy, MD, Series Editor
Mini-textbooks in question-and-answer format to help students, residents, and practitioners hone their skills for practice and board exams.

- CRITICAL CARE SECRETS, by Polly E. Parsons, MD, and Jeanine P. Wiener-Kronish, MD, 1992, $32.95

- EMERGENCY MEDICINE SECRETS, by Vince Markovchick, MD, Peter Pons, MD, and Richard Wolfe, MD, 1993, $30.00

- MEDICAL SECRETS, by Anthony J. Zollo, Jr., MD, 1991, $33.95

- NEUROLOGY SECRETS, by Loren A. Rolak, MD, 1993, $32.00

- OB/GYN SECRETS, by Helen L. Frederickson, MD, and Louise Wilkins-Haug, MD, 1991, $28.95

- PEDIATRIC SECRETS, by Richard A. Polin, MD, and Mark F. Ditmar, MD, 1989, $30.95

- SURGICAL SECRETS, 2nd ed., by Charles M. Abernathy, MD, and Alden H. Harken, MD, 1991, $29.95

DEDICATION

To Hans,

     In loving memory,

          Rosie

To my wife Kathleen Sewell Meador, whose tolerance, support, and love endured the writing of this book.

       C.K.M.

INTRODUCTION

Clifton K. Meador, M.D.

Nurses and doctors have had an interdependent relationship for a long time. While some may disagree, neither profession can function comprehensively without the other. The contents of this book and the process of its creation illustrate this collaborative and interdependent relationship between doctors and nurses.

There are rules that are specific and peculiar only to the practice of medicine. These are detailed in the companion book, *A Little Book of Doctors' Rules.** We omitted all rules

---

* Meador CK: A Little Book of Doctors' Rules. Philadelphia, Hanley & Belfus, 1992.

particular to the practice of medicine from the present book. However, there are rules of human communication and conduct that overlap and are common to medicine and nursing. Such rules apply to all professions if not all people. They are called common courtesy. The essence of these overlapping rules, as pertinent to nursing, are repeated.

There are two other general types of rules—those that describe appropriate behaviors between doctors and nurses and those that are peculiar to the nursing profession. Only a nurse can describe the latter. When our publisher Linda Belfus first suggested the idea of A Book of Nurses' Rules, I immediately thought of Rosalie Hammerschmidt, R.N.

Rosalie Hammerschmidt's unique nursing experiences make her an ideal coauthor. She was a pioneer in critical care nursing in the early 1960s at Presbyterian Hospital in Pittsburgh where she worked with Dr. Peter Safar, the renowned critical care specialist. She was one of the founders of the American Association of Critical Care Nurses (AACN) and served on the board of directors and as the organization's national president in 1973. Her most passionate dream was for doctors and nurses to coauthor and publish articles in the same scientific journal. Her dream was realized during her AACN Presidency when *Heart and Lung*, now the *American Journal of Critical Care*, began publication. She was honored in 1975 with a term as Nurse Editor of the unique journal she championed.

Rosalie Hammerschmidt has made major contributions to critical care nursing as a clinician, educator, and nursing leader. She played a significant role in the establishment, evolution, and acceptance of prehospital emergency care in Nashville and was widely respected for her teaching of paramedics both in the classroom and under the rigors of field conditions. She was deeply involved in quality assurance and utilization of clinical resources in patient care both at Vanderbilt University Hospital and Saint Thomas Hospital.

For several years she and I practiced together in a referral and consulting practice of endocrinology and internal medicine. During that period we uncovered many of the rules in this book and in the companion book, *A Little Book of Doctors' Rules.* It is a privilege to join her in writing this book.

Some people are put off by the whole notion of rules. It is our contention that all behavior is driven by rules, mostly unstated and implicit. It is our intent to make some of these rules explicit so we can begin to distinguish those rules that are important from those that are not. We could not resist including some lesser rules that describe the humorous side of nursing. Although nurses and doctors work in a serious profession, we do not have to take ourselves too seriously. We trust we have not offended too many with these lighter approaches.

In *A Little Book of Doctors' rules*, I described three essential elements of a good rule. These were:

"*First*, a good rule makes intuitive sense. It has a ring of truth.

Second, a valid rule has been observed to be helpful in its application or harmful in its violation.

Third, a sound rule is stated in a manner that allows affirmation or refutation by direct, systematic observation of others. This last consideration fulfills the essential potential for being scientific."

We hope the rules in this book meet these requirements.

PREFACE

Rosalie Hammerschmidt, R.N.

This is a little book about nurses, both our serious and our lighter sides. It contains rules about our practice styles, our patients, our colleagues, our profession, and mostly about ourselves.

While working on this book, I drew extensively from my years of active nursing practice, even remembering sometimes the specific situation or person I associated with a rule. This occurrence made writing the rules a pleasure. I hope you will also have similar pleasant experiences as you read the book.

Of all the rules I've written, the ones I value the most are those that come from when I was a patient in the hospital. The common theme that connects this special group of rules has to do with honesty, respect, dignity, privacy, and autonomy—in short *personhood*.

Writing the rules was a beneficial experience in several ways. As I read and reread the manuscript, I took an honest and thoughtful look at my personal and professional life. Three beliefs I have about nursing were strongly reaffirmed. First, that a nurse's attitudes and behaviors have a profound effect upon a patient's health and well-being. Further, that learning and practicing the art of nursing is a challenging and worthwhile pursuit. Lastly, that nurses and physicians should focus time and energy on the areas of their practice that are similar and complementary. This is essential if we are to foster the collaboration that ultimately benefits the patients we serve.

I hope you enjoy the rules and take the time to send in any of your own for inclusion in the next edition. A suggestion form is provided at the end of the book.

ACKNOWLEDGMENTS

Rosalie Hammerschmidt, R.N.

This book is a reality because of Clifton Meador, M.D., who graciously invited me to join him as coauthor of *A Little Book of Nurses' Rules.* I am grateful to Dr. Meador for his elegance as a physician and as a person. He approaches everyone he meets with kindness and respect and in so doing creates a therapeutic environment of acceptance and concern. I owe him special gratitude for the twenty years of our professional association in which he freely shared his academic brilliance, compassionate humanity, gracious generosity, and contagious good humor. I hold in high regard Dr. Meador's belief that patients receive the best possible care when physicians and nurses work together in the spirit of mutual respect and trust. This book is the result of our collaborative effort.

I am grateful to my teachers, colleagues, and friends at Presbyterian Hospital in Pittsburgh for providing me the solid foundation of knowledge and skills to start my nursing career. I am especially indebted to Dr. Peter Safar, my mentor and friend, who taught me to appreciate the interrelatedness of body systems when making clinical decisions and the subtleties of the early recognition and treatment of hypoxia. Both these lessons have served me well and have been the cornerstone of my clinical practice. To Dr. Leonard Caccamo for teaching me electrophysiology and bedside diagnosis of the cardiac patient, I owe my gratitude.

I extend warmest thanks to my friends and colleagues for reading the early drafts, making suggestions, and offering encouragement. These special people include Joyce Pareigis RN,

Mitzi Sprouse RN, Mary Wicker RN, Nina Jeffords RN, Penny Vaughan RN, Joy Smith RN, Sister Almeda Golson DC, Sister Colette Hanlon SC, Don Moore PhD, Virginia Fuqua, Reba Barrett RN, and Susan Jackson.

I owe special thanks to Jan Dunn RN and Carolee Hardin PT for the rules they shared and their untiring encouragement and support.

I extend my heartfelt gratitude and appreciation to the thousands of folks whom I have cared for over the past thirty years. You taught me the important things about life that cannot be learned from a book or a lecture.

THERE IS NO RULE WITHOUT AN EXCEPTION.
MOST RULES CAN BE BROKEN.

1   Sit down when you talk with patients.

whether it is a nursing history,
a patient education session,
or discharge instructions.

2   The good nurse knows what she does not know.

3   There is no blood or urine test to measure mental function.
There probably never will be.

| 4 | Learn to do a thorough mental status evaluation. |

Do it as you go along.

Fill it in later.

    mood,
    affect,
    attitude,
    appearance,
    disorganized vs. organized,
    rapport,
    speech content,
    delusions, hallucinations,
    judgment,
    memory, recent and remote.

| 5 | Be wary of patients who are overly complimentary of you as a nurse, especially on first meetings.

An E.R. stretcher is sticking out in the hallway.

The emergency code cart is covered with EKG paper and empty syringes, and all drawers are open.

You meet a city policeman on the elevator who asks directions to your unit.

A nurse is filling out 3 incident reports

Bloody sheets and pillows are flowing into the hallway from a patient's room.

The head nurse is asking in a loud voice if anyone wants overtime.

| 7 | Reflex hammers and stethoscopes disappear. |

| 8 | Most people are healthy and will live long lives. |

| 9 | Always examine the part that the patient complains about. Put your hand on the area. |

| 10 | The only way to determine a patient's needs is to:
listen,
look carefully, and
ask good questions. |

| 11 | Watch patients carefully who are being treated with a second drug to correct a reaction to a first drug. |

12 No suppository belongs in the nose.

13 When patients are admitted to the hospital, they bring their dignity with them.

Make sure no one robs them of it.

14 False teeth get lost.

15 Touch patients each time you see them, even if you only hold their hands or feel the pulse.

Do this especially with older people.

Caution:
Some patients prefer to reach out and touch you first.

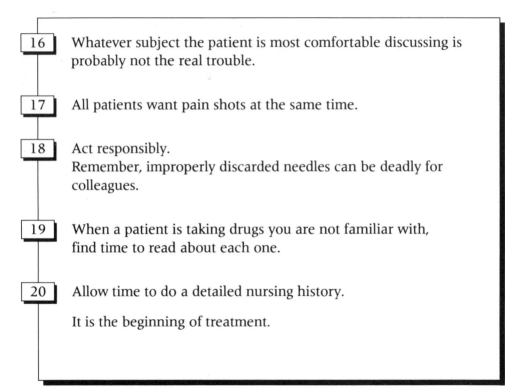

16 Whatever subject the patient is most comfortable discussing is probably not the real trouble.

17 All patients want pain shots at the same time.

18 Act responsibly.
Remember, improperly discarded needles can be deadly for colleagues.

19 When a patient is taking drugs you are not familiar with, find time to read about each one.

20 Allow time to do a detailed nursing history.

It is the beginning of treatment.

| 21 | Do not let stress compromise your practice.
If you even remotely suspect it is:
    step back,
    take an inventory of yourself,
    and change something.

. . . anything.

You change and the world around you changes.

| 22 | Base your choice of where to practice nursing on:

    the philosophy of the organization,
    the standards of nursing practice,
    the strength of the nursing department to effect policy,
    and the opportunity to pursue your career path.

Slick ads showing photographs of nurses on beaches do not
speak to any of these.

| 23 | Read *A Short Life of Florence Nightingale*.* |

| 24 | Help nurses who "float" to your unit. |
| | Try to keep their heads above water. |

Do not let them sink.

| 25 | Do not get your drug information exclusively from the *PDR*. |

Follow current literature and check drug alert bulletins monthly.

| 26 | TWO TYPES OF ADHESIVE TAPE |

The kind that will not stick.
The kind that will not come off.

* Nash R: A Short Life of Florence Nightingale. New York, Macmillan Company, 1931.

27 You must give permission to enable a patient to discuss unusual or deviant behaviors. Do this in a very specific manner:

If you think a patient may be abusing some drug, say, "Some people take only a tablespoon of milk of magnesia a day, some take 2 or 3 bottles a day. How much do you take?"

28 If your dislike of a patient (or anyone for that matter) is severe, the patient either has a serious personality disorder

or

he or she may be acting out an aspect of yourself that you despise or disown.

29 Being a nurse is a privilege.
Do not abuse it.

It is easy to forget this rule in times of stress . . .
particularly when you are busy and your patient's needs become great.

30

Just as soon after a workday as possible, take time to review the day.

> Celebrate the good things that happened,
> Decide what you could have done differently or better.
> Then let it all go and relax.

31

If a patient's room smells bad to you, it will smell awful to the patient and the family.

Change it.

32

Hospital policies are only guidelines.

They cover about 90% of what we do.
Use common sense in handling the other 10%.
Policies, like rules, have exceptions.

33 Being assertive is not being aggressive.
Learn the difference.

Assertiveness reflects a positive self-image.
It is the foundation of good communication.

Aggressiveness reflects frustration and anger.
It is counterproductive when dealing with people.

34 Respect everyone you meet, especially those who work in
supportive jobs in the hospital.

They make it possible for you to be an effective nurse.

35 I.V. stands are at the opposite end of the hall when you need
them most.

36 Make certain that you know as much about life and people as you do about physiology, biochemistry, and anatomy.

Let your patients and others teach you.

37 Set goals **with** a patient rather than **for** a patient.
After all, the patient is the one who is trying to meet the goals.

38 As a nurse, your odds are high for:

committing suicide,
getting divorced,
becoming addicted,
being co-dependent, or
going off the deep end.

Find out why.

39 Read the book *I'm Dying to Take Care of You* by Candace Snow and David Willard.*

40 Know those things you can change.

Know those things you cannot change.

Develop the wisdom to tell the difference.

41 Learn to say "No" tactfully.

Just say "No."

42 Say "No" at least once every day.

* Snow C, Willard D: I'm Dying to Take Care of You. Redmond, WA, Professional Counseling Books, 1989.

43 Technology has provided us with new mechanical devices to prevent bedsores.

Their benefit is finite.

There is no substitute for meticulous, manual skin care in patients at high risk.

44 A patient's resistance to receiving therapy needs to be respected, listened to, and dealt with.

45 If you do not like nursing, get out of it today.

46 There is no such thing as an uninteresting patient.
People are all fascinating in some way.
Discover what that is.

| 47 | A detailed drug history includes over-the-counter drugs.

The average person's medicine cabinet is filled with drugs. When is the last time you looked in yours?

| 48 | There is no such thing as an organ-specific drug. All drugs work throughout the body.

| 49 | Never ask the patient, "How are **we** doing?"

You should already know how **you** are doing.

| 50 | Do not tell a patient, "There is nothing wrong with you."

It is demeaning and insulting.

| 51 | Learn something from every patient you meet.

52 The only acceptable color of a stain on a sheet is white.

Remove all others immediately.

53 When you are listening to a patient, do not do anything else.

Just listen.

54 The admitting office puts all patients with identical names on the same unit.

Whenever possible, they put them in the same room.

55 Citizenship is important.
Get involved in your community, your schools, your government.

56
Some diseases are not treatable,
but all patients can be given care.

57
Patient's families who are angry or hostile are reacting to
something . . . real or perceived.

Establish rapport and hear them out.
Designate one nurse to follow the situation and avoid confusion.

58
No person ever arrives in the emergency room wearing
his or her best underwear.

59
Learn how the intestine functions.
It is the first step in preventing constipation and fecal
impactions.

You will never be sorry.
Your patients will thank you.

| 60 | If you are in academic nursing, take time out each year to work in a practice setting where you give direct patient care. |

| 61 | Learn one area of nursing in great depth. It will give you respect for scientific knowledge and nursing research. |

| 62 | Choose and buy the standard textbook in your nursing specialty.

Buy the latest edition whenever it is published.

Do this for the rest of your career. |

| 63 | Subscribe to your nursing specialty journal **now**. If you do not read it, at least scan it. Do this for the rest of your career. |

64 Organize a journal club to review current literature.
You will learn much and enjoy your colleagues at the same time.

65 There are only three ways to answer a question:
I don't know, but I'll find out.
I don't know, but I'll guess.
I know.

66 If routine practice does not meet the patient's needs . . .
change the *routine*.

67 Remember learning medical terminology?
Most of your patients never took that class.
Be certain they understand what you are trying to tell them.

Encourage questions.
Answer respectfully.
Never sound condescending.

68 Many patients do not understand milligrams, milliliters, centimeters, or even ounces.

Use terms they understand and be sure the measuring device is in the units they will use at home.

69 Food and liquids do not belong in the lung.

70 The weight and height tables are not verities.
There are tall people and there are short people.
There are heavy people and there are thin people.
There are endomorphs, ectomorphs, and mesomorphs.
Everybody has to be one thing or another.

71 When you meet a patient for the first time, allow a few minutes for the patient to tell you what is on his or her mind.

You will learn a lot.

| 72 | Do not write in the chart and talk with a patient at the same time. |

| 73 | If you make a mistake in treatment, acknowledge it immediately. Your patient's welfare depends on it. |

| 74 | Develop a list of nurses you trust and respect, nurture your relationship with them, and call them when you need their advice. |

| 75 | Learn what collaborative practice is.

Nurses and doctors share the responsibility for patient care. |

| 76 | Make your voice heard.

Your nursing organization can represent you only if you are an active part of it. |

| 77 | We all have a unique way of expressing our thoughts. Adjust your thinking to the patient's pace and style. |

| 78 | Listen for what the patient is **not** telling you. |

| 79 | Time is distorted when waiting for:
a doctor or nurse,
news of a loved one,
the report of an important test,
a biopsy result, and
pain medicine. |

| 80 | One or even several days on a regular diet is not going to kill someone on a low-cholesterol diet.

You will, however, have to deal with some patients who believe that even one meal off their diet is lethal. |

| 81 | Check on the legal status of incident reports in your hospital and in your state.

Be careful what you write and how you write it.
Be accurate.
Be factual.
Be scrupulously honest.

Remember, your incident reports can make very good plaintiff reading from the witness stand.

| 82 | The best defenses against malpractice are:
complete honesty,
clinical vigilance,
clinical knowledge and skill,
a well-documented clinical record, and
careful communication between all members of the care
team, between nurses, and between the care team and the
patient and the family.

83　If you are involved in a malpractice suit, be very careful before you accuse someone else of giving poor care.

Remember, plaintiff attorneys are doing everything possible to pit one member of the care team against another.

84　Never appear shocked by anything a patient tells you.

85　It is all right for a patient to
　　cry,
　　get depressed,
　　laugh,
　　hurt,
　　or have any other feeling.

86　It is all right for a patient to get angry.

87 Do not talk to an angry patient about any other subject until you understand the source of the anger.

Take as long as necessary to diffuse the anger.

88 There is no external method to measure the presence or absence of pain.

89 There is no external method to measure how much pain a patient is having.

90 A watched I.V. bag never runs out.

91 Never make an assumption about a drug dosage.

If you or others cannot read a doctor's handwriting, call the doctor and ask.

92 Intake and output are vital bits of clinical information. Measure carefully and accurately.

93 A dehydrated patient remains dehydrated until total accumulated fluid intake significantly exceeds accumulated output.

If accumulated intake does not exceed accumulated output in a dehydrated patient after a few hours, call the physician. The patient needs a higher rate of intravenous fluids.

94 Severely dehydrated patients with diabetes mellitus can make large amounts of urine per hour.

Just because a patient is making a large hourly volume of urine does not mean you are gaining on the dehydration.

This false assumption is a common source of error.

| 95 | Any new abnormality that occurs with the addition of a new drug is due to the drug until proved otherwise. |

| 96 | The absence of a reported specific toxicity of a drug does not mean it cannot or does not occur. |

| 97 | Drug reactions can be unique to a single patient. |

| 98 | There is no manifestation that cannot be caused by any given drug.

or

Any drug can do anything. |

| 99 | There are no controlled studies of patients taking more than four drugs and very few of patients taking three.

Any patient on more than four drugs is beyond medical science. |

| 100 | The likelihood of an adverse drug reaction rises exponentially with an increase in the number of drugs administered.

| 101 | The good nursing supervisor:

is calm, cool, and collected no matter what,
can retrieve false teeth from a burning incinerator,
can find keys to every room in the hospital,
can start impossible I.V.s with one attempt,
can find lost wedding rings in contaminated needle
    containers,
can make combative patients think she is a close relative,
    and
can leap up or down four flights of stairs in emergencies and
    not get short of breath.

| 102 | Use the English language correctly and concisely.

| 103 | Never say irregardless. |

| 104 | Tincture of time is frequently the best medicine. |

| 105 | Superior nurses know the sequence of what is important. |

| 106 | Do not get in a chart-writing fight with doctors or anyone else. Chart fights do not make good reading from the witness stand. |

| 107 | Insist on reading verbal orders back to the physician. |

| 108 | Never point or shake your finger at a patient. If you do that, please stop it. |

| 109 | If a person's eyes are constantly moving as you talk, he or she is not listening with full attention. |

110 The first step in effective communication is to gain the full attention of the other person.
Sometimes this requires long periods of silence.

111 It is impossible to think and listen simultaneously.
Listen
Think
Listen
Think

112 Listening requires practice.

Learn to stop thinking.
Learn to listen.

Just listen.

113 Laughter among nurses attracts supervisors and directors of nursing.

| 114 | The major concern of the nurse is to know the person with the disease as a person. |

| 115 | Do not tolerate arrogant or condescending behavior. |

Not in physicians.
Not in fellow nurses,
Not in administrators,
Not in coworkers from other departments,
Not in patients,
Not in anyone.

Find a way and the right time to confront these behaviors constructively.

Remember, timing is everything in life.

| 116 | Do not call physicians for laxative orders after midnight. Few doctors are interested in a patient's bowel habits after dark. |

117 Avoid "organ" talk.

Do not ask
"How is your colon?"
or
"Your stomach?"
or
"Your sinuses?"
or
"Your heart?"
or
any other organ.

Ask how the patient feels.

Do not let patients use organ talk.
Only patients know how they feel or what they think.
Insist on a language of symptoms, feelings, and thoughts.

| 118 | If you do not like the behavior of another person, consider changing **your** behavior.

| 119 | If you find yourself being frequently surprised by the responses of patients, you may be sending multiple messages:

> One message with your words . . .
>
> A different message with your tone of voice . . .
>
> Another with your facial expression . . .
>
> Still another with your body posture . . .
>
> Only an audio-video tape of yourself will uncover this kind of problem.

| 120 | The nurse must interact with all people in a hospital.
Only nurses, CEOs, and COOs must do that.

121 The essentials of the nursing process are:

Assess
Plan
Implement
Evaluate
Revise plan

These steps are repeated until the patient is discharged.

122 The occupation of your patient is important clinically.
Know what it is.
Learn something about it.
Over the years you will learn a lot.

123 The error of unrecognized dementia in hospitalized patients is common.

Cognitive mental status evaluations are too often omitted.

124 | The social persona is the last thing to be lost in dementia. Do not be fooled by its preservation.

It does not take much brain power to be pleasant, sociable, or carry on a rambling but polite conversation.

Or even to act like the chairman of the board.

125 | Patients with early dementia will do everything possible to hide their disorientation.

They will even read dates from nearby milk cartons or newspapers if tested for orientation.

126 | Assessment of orientation to time must include the day of the week, the date of the month, the month, and **the year**.

Orientation to time in early dementia can remain intact to everything except **the year**.

THE RESPONSE YOU GET IS THE MESSAGE YOU SEND

If a patient gets mad as you talk,
you said something that angered the patient.

If a patient laughs as you talk,
you said something that was funny to the patient.

If the patient cries as you talk,
you said something that was sad or upsetting to the patient.

If the patient begins to argue with you,
you said something argumentative to the patient.

You can be in charge of your communication.

Do not tolerate doctors who throw instruments or charts.

Find the time to confront this behavior in an assertive, positive
way.

129	Two patients in a room make four times the work of one.
130	Speak so you can be heard.
131	Write so others can read it.
132	Wash your hands before you touch a patient. Do it in front of your patients.
133	There are few drugs as relaxing as a good back rub.
134	Bed baths attract visitors, families, and physicians on teaching rounds.

| 135 | Enemas, sedatives, and use of multiple drugs cause nighttime falls.

Be on extra alert with such patients.

| 136 | Patients who get serious injuries with falls in hospitals often have already had a previous fall on the same admission.

After the first fall, get a family member or someone to stay with the patient at all times.

| 137 | Post DRUG ALLERGY ALERTS in as many places as possible.

| 138 | Always check for a DRUG ALLERGY ALERT before giving any drug.

139 Integrity is your most valuable asset.
Never compromise it.

140 Do not try to move patients who weigh more than 300 pounds
by yourself, especially if they are wedged in the shower stall.

141 Do not leave the room while the patient is talking.
If necessary, interrupt the patient and explain why you are
leaving.

142 Always observe the patient walking.

143 No organ system fails in isolation.
Be aware of this when developing a nursing care plan.

144 Weight gain or loss within 7 days is all water.

145 Do not stereotype people.

146 Alcohol on the breath does not necessarily mean the patient is intoxicated,

nor does it necessarily mean that the patient is an alcoholic.

147 Never tell a patient, "Don't worry."

148 Talk *with*, not *to* patients.

149 Take time to show your appreciation to others.

150 Never fail to praise others for jobs well done.

151 Keep an open mind.

New ideas become available to you when you do.

152 Attend your nursing school reunions.

153 A person is not a "diabetic" but a unique human being who can strive to live a full and productive life while coping with a disease—diabetes mellitus.

154 A hospital is a dangerous place.

It should be used wisely and as briefly as possible.

155 It is a human impossibility to have all the information
you will need when you call a physician.
At least have the chart in hand when you do call.

156 Always remember that restlessness may mean hypoxemia.
Evaluate the patient carefully before giving any sedation.

157 Weigh every patient on admission to the hospital.
If patients are on intravenous fluids, weigh them every day.

158 Never wake a patient to give a sedative, analgesic, or laxative.

159 A nurse who treats herself has a fool for a patient.

Remember, you are a role model for others on matters
of health.

160
If a man pulls out a Foley catheter with a 5 c.c. bag, he may just be frustrated and upset.

If he pulls out a Foley with a 30 c.c. bag, do a mental status assessment.

161
Always introduce yourself to your patients.

Name tags are difficult to read,
especially when the patient is very sick and without glasses.

162
Ask patients with chronic symptoms two questions:
    What are you doing that you should stop doing?
    What are you not doing that you should be doing?

163
Always make rounds with physicians.
This rule is frequently violated.
It should not be.

164 | The best treatment plan comes when the patient, the doctor, and the nurse are in the same place at the same time.

This rule is also frequently violated.

It should not be.

165 | The one mark of a professional nurse:
Commit yourself to give the highest possible quality care to all of your patients.

166 | Good communication means "getting through."

Good communication is not merely "talking to" another person.

167 | First, think of the easy.

168 When you hear hoofbeats on a bridge, think first of a horse, not a zebra.

169 Assume that unconscious patients (including those anesthetized) hear, understand, and will remember what you are saying.

170 Reserve resuscitation for witnessed cardiac arrests.

If your hospital has a policy that opposes this, try to get it changed.

171 Do not steal narcotics.

In fact, do not steal.

172 Suspect physical abuse when the story does not fit the injury.

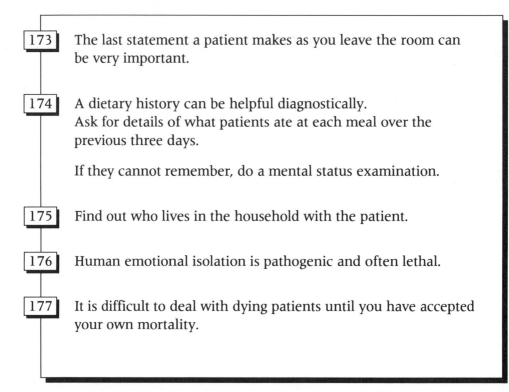

173   The last statement a patient makes as you leave the room can be very important.

174   A dietary history can be helpful diagnostically.
Ask for details of what patients ate at each meal over the previous three days.

If they cannot remember, do a mental status examination.

175   Find out who lives in the household with the patient.

176   Human emotional isolation is pathogenic and often lethal.

177   It is difficult to deal with dying patients until you have accepted your own mortality.

178 Balance in life is essential to well-being.
Pursue a hobby or some interest outside nursing.

179 Do yourself a favor.
Always take your vacations.
Get out of town.

180 The higher the technology, the greater the need for human touch.

181 Your personal qualities as a nurse can be as important therapeutically as any drug or treatment.

182 After midnight, all cases get clinically strange.

183 Do not gossip.

184 The best way to know the effect your words have on another
person is to watch his or her face as you speak.

185 Notice the change in respiratory rate as you discuss different
subjects with patients.

Watch the top edge of the shoulder.
It rises with each inhalation.

186 Get to know the patient's family.
The time is well spent.

187 Make the patient's family an ally, not the enemy.

188 All disease labels are abstractions.

Only the patient is concrete.

189 Do not back out of the room as you are talking with the patient.

190 Eat lunch with people with positive attitudes.
Do not even drink coffee with those with negative attitudes.

191 Be wary of the patient who walks out of an ambulance into the emergency room and announces he could not afford taxi fare.

192 People like to sleep at night.

193 Learn to work **with** not **against** the housestaff.

They can be fun.
They can teach you some things.
You can teach them some things.
Everybody learns.

194 Do not discuss your personal life with patients,
especially your love life or sexual life.

If you feel an urge to do that, make some new or different
friends or reconnect with your family.

195 There is a direct correlation between the difficulty in starting
an I.V. and the clinical need for it.

196 Learn the difference between "informed persuasion" and
"informed consent."

| 197 | If you do something three times and it does not work, chances are the next time you do it . . . it will not work. |

| 198 | There is an unconscious mind. |

| 199 | Never ignore an experienced nurse's observation. |

| 200 | Listen very carefully when a patient prefaces a comment with, "This may not be important, but . . ." |

| 201 | Never forget:

Being a patient can be demeaning and frightening.
Frightened and demeaned people will exhibit almost any kind of behavior.

It is your job as a nurse to minimize fear and anxiety. |

| 202 | If the sterility of an object is suspect . . . it is unsterile. |

| 203 | Be wary of people who bring a sterling silver cover for the hospital telephone receiver. |

| 204 | Be wary of seductive patients.
Learn how to deal with them in a straightforward manner. |

| 205 | Never, ever, have a sexual relationship with a patient. |

| 206 | Be alert for hypnotic-sedative abuse, especially in older people.

Withdrawal symptoms such as a seizure may be your first clue. |

| 207 | Respect your nursing colleagues and develop a network with those nurses you admire.

They will add richness and vitality to your professional life. |

208 Allow enough time to do a thorough assessment of the patient. Include the following functions:

> biophysical,
> social,
> psychological,
> spiritual, and
> cultural.

209 The information in the nursing history is the foundation for a nursing plan that will work for the whole patient.

210 When dealing with depressed patients, remember there is often repressed anger.

211 Explain to patients who are taking antidepressants why they must take the drug all the time, not just when they feel depressed.

212 There is an unfortunate trend toward team bathing of patients.

No one wants to be bathed by a gang.

Group washings should be reserved for public swimming pools, car washes, and visits to Japan.

213 There is no substitute for direct observation.

214 There is no substitute for data.

215 Measure, measure, measure.
Observe, observe, observe.

216 Sedate patients with caution.

Confusion or restlessness can be caused by a multitude of physiologic states.

Fever, hypoglycemia, and hypoxia come to mind first.

217 | Before asking the physician for a sedation order:

First, rule out physiologic causes in which sedation is contraindicated.

Then ask yourself:

Is this sedative to benefit me?
   or
Is it to benefit the patient?

This is a hard question to ask yourself . . . but it is important.

218 | The best prevention for malpractice is rapport with the patient and complete honesty.

219 | Someone needs to invent a warm bedpan.

220 | Human perfection is an oxymoron.

221 General questions produce informative answers.

"Can you tell me about your breathing?"

The patient will tell his or her story.

Specific questions produce limited information.

"Have you ever had any shortness of breath?"

The patient can only respond "yes" or "no."

222 Physical restraint of patients substitutes one set of problems for another . . .

patient safety from the restraints themselves,
skin breakdown, and
anxiety of family and friends, to name a few.

223 Take your job seriously.
Your patients deserve the best.

224 Take yourself lightly.
You deserve the best.

225 Laughter is a natural tranquilizer.

It is free,
nonfattening,
salt free,
without side effects,
and available for use by anyone.

Best of all, it is contagious.

226 When you give instructions, ask the patient to repeat what you have said.

227 It is not necessary to speak in a loud voice to patients on ventilators.

| 228 | Be aware of and sensitive to the elderly's natural losses:

> decreased hearing, poor appetite, loss of eyesight, difficulty sleeping, bowel irregularity.

Be sensitive to their psychological needs and symptoms:

> loneliness, depression, fear of being a burden, fear of death, loss of spouse, loss of friends, debilitation.

| 229 | A map of a territory is not the same as the territory.
Do not confuse a model of reality with reality.

| 230 | Imagine how you would feel if you were very sick, half naked in a short ill-fitting gown, and abandoned in a strange environment.

Remember that feeling when you are caring for your patients.

231

The normal limits for laboratory tests are not verities.
They are only statistically derived and defined terms.

Remember, there are at least 2.5% of the public who live
healthy and long lives above the upper limits of any test.

Also remember, there are at least 2.5% of the public who live
healthy and long lives below the lower limits of any test.

Everybody has to be somewhere.

232

When you call a physician during the night, make certain it is
a genuine request for help or serious concern about a patient's
status.

If not, everything else can wait until morning.

233

Occasionally you can disarm a difficult patient with a
compliment and make him or her your ally.

| 234 | You are not going to change anyone's eating habits during a hospital stay.

When you instruct hospitalized patients about their diets:

Go easy.
Be reasonable.
Use common sense.

| 235 | Use it or lose it.
This rule applies to all parts of the body.

| 236 | A loud voice will not penetrate:

total nerve deafness,
mental confusion,
or unconsciousness.

Yelling will not translate English into Spanish.

237 | Every system of health care should be patient centered.

238 | Each nurse has the same properties as a drug.

With each encounter, his or her actions can:

produce side effects
exhibit a duration of action
induce toxicity
be indicated
be contraindicated
be given in an overdose
be given in an underdose
be given at the right interval
be given at the wrong interval
or most commonly

produce a placebo effect.

Learn the pharmacology of being a nurse.

239 Patients frequently do not take drugs as prescribed.

240 For most internal emotional states there is a visible and
audible external representation in the face, body,
and/or voice.

The astute observer learns to see and hear this.

241 DRUG ABUSE

No one is well served by ignoring a drug-abusing colleague.

Not you,
not your colleague,
and above all, not your patients.

Find out what you should do if you are certain a colleague is
abusing drugs.

Then do it.

242 | If you instruct a patient to take medicines at certain times, be sure the patient can tell time.

Also be sure the patient has a watch.

243 | Tell people approaching old age:

"Never start taking short steps."

It is a habit that can be avoided.

244 | Do not hasten death.
Do not prolong it needlessly.

245 | About the time you think you have seen it all, you will encounter some new unbelievable behavior.

There is no limit to the endless variety of human behavior.

246 Any tube inserted into a major orifice should be firmly secured to the skin with tape.

No one wants:
a wiggling nasogastric tube,
a flopping endotracheal tube, or
someone stepping on the tubing from the Foley catheter.

247 Many people confuse the terms "life expectancy" with "human life span."

Learn the difference.

248 Never refer to patients with pejorative terms like "crock," "shad," "turkey," or "gomer."

It only reveals your inability to understand the world of the other person.

It is also rude and unprofessional.

249 Assume that no one has ever been a patient in a hospital before.

Even if the patient is a doctor or nurse.

250 Jails and hospitals have many similarities.
They are the only two public institutions that:

> take away clothing and issue uniforms,
> remove valuables and personal belongings,
> allow visiting on a limited basis,
> assign people to rooms with complete strangers,
> designate people only by numbers,
> prohibit freedom of movement, and
> serve very limited kinds of food.

Try to minimize all other similarities.

You are the patient's nurse, not his warden.

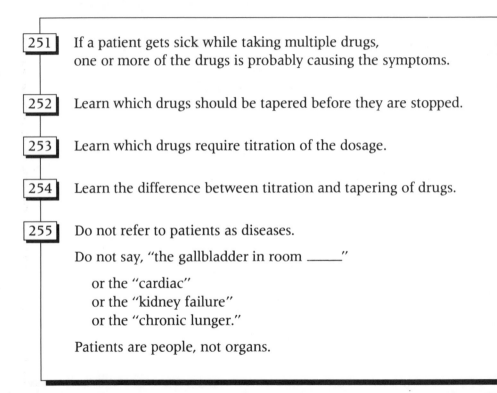

251 If a patient gets sick while taking multiple drugs,
one or more of the drugs is probably causing the symptoms.

252 Learn which drugs should be tapered before they are stopped.

253 Learn which drugs require titration of the dosage.

254 Learn the difference between titration and tapering of drugs.

255 Do not refer to patients as diseases.

Do not say, "the gallbladder in room _____"

　　or the "cardiac"
　　or the "kidney failure"
　　or the "chronic lunger."

Patients are people, not organs.

256 A bed bath may be just a nursing task to you, but to your patients it is a highly personal and intimate experience.

257 Use the time in giving a bed bath to:

    do a complete physical assessment,
    offer reassurance,
    do patient education,
    assess mental function,
    answer questions,
    build rapport,
    and maybe to get the patient to smile.

258 Always be careful of hysterical patients.
They can have several diseases.

259 The less often a patient has to take a medicine,
the more likely he is to take each dose.

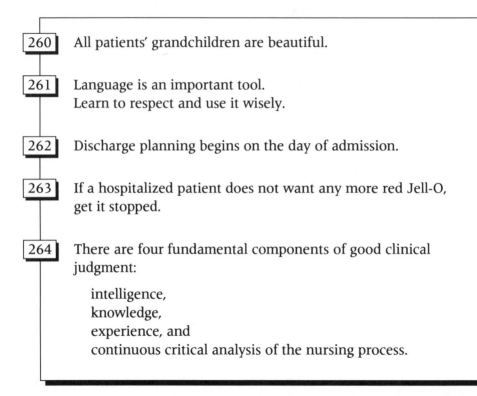

260 All patients' grandchildren are beautiful.

261 Language is an important tool.
Learn to respect and use it wisely.

262 Discharge planning begins on the day of admission.

263 If a hospitalized patient does not want any more red Jell-O, get it stopped.

264 There are four fundamental components of good clinical judgment:

intelligence,
knowledge,
experience, and
continuous critical analysis of the nursing process.

265 Unfortunately, our entire system of care too often teaches patients to stay sick, not to get well.

266 Patients are sometimes labeled as "difficult."
Usually the problem is the nurse who finds it **difficult** to know how to treat them.

Do not miss the chance to learn from such situations.
These patients have much to teach us about ourselves.

267 As soon as you are gloved and gowned, the itching will begin.

268 Confusion can be an essential phase of the learning process.

269 Pay careful attention to patients who say they are going to die.

270 The first clue of early dementia may be confusion at night.

271 Never ask a patient to do a favor for you.

272 Teach patients to be well, not sick.

273 Never take away hope.

274 When you do not know what you are doing,

STOP!

275 Do know harm.

Do no harm.

276 Use knowledge as a tool to improve your life and those around you.

Never use it as a weapon to intimidate others.

277 Patients are not diseases.
They are people who are afflicted with a disease.

278 Rule for Calculating Time for Completion of a Procedure:

Multiply the physician's estimated time by 1.3 and add 19.

279 Teach patients to live the highest quality of life possible in spite of their illness.

280 FIVE RIGHTS OF GIVING MEDICATIONS

1. The right DRUG
2. The right DOSE
3. The right ROUTE
4. The right TIME

     and

5. THE RIGHT PATIENT

281 All of the known drug interactions are probably only a small percent of the total.

282 Read the label of all medications three times:

ONCE . . . before removing the container from the drawer or shelf

ONCE . . . before removing the drug from the container

ONCE . . . upon returning the container to the drawer or shelf

283 Teach the patient to develop and use a self-rating scale from 0 to 10 to chart the progress of symptoms.

This is particularly helpful in following patients with pain.

284 Stories and metaphors are wonderful teaching devices. To be effective they must be closely related to the life and world of the patient.

There are three kinds of patients.

1. Those who believe every word you say and do everything you suggest.

   Be careful what you say and suggest.

2. Those who reflect on what you say, wonder why you said it, ask you questions, and then make up their own minds about what they do.

   Answer all their questions.

3. Those who disagree with everything you say, oppose every suggestion you make, and state that nothing will help them.

   Preface every suggestion you make by saying that the suggestion may or may not work.

Learn to deal with all three kinds of patients.

286 Learning to deal with bedpans while preserving personal and patient dignity is the mark of a real nurse.

287 A few patients seem to be saying, "I want you to help me but I will not let you."

288 Someone needs to invent a homing device to find lost false teeth.

289 Incident reports . . .

When in doubt, fill one out.

290 Ignored and abandoned families and patients become frightened and angry.

Angry and frightened people sue.

291 An axiom of charting . . .

"Not charted" equals "not done."

292 You are the patient's advocate.

Your nursing practice should reflect the trust patients place in you.

293 Learn the difference between the words multidisciplinary and interdisciplinary.

When you do: collaboration, team conference, and care planning take on new meanings.

294 Be sure you know as much about the patient clinically as you do about his laboratory numbers.

Remember, numbers come from real people.

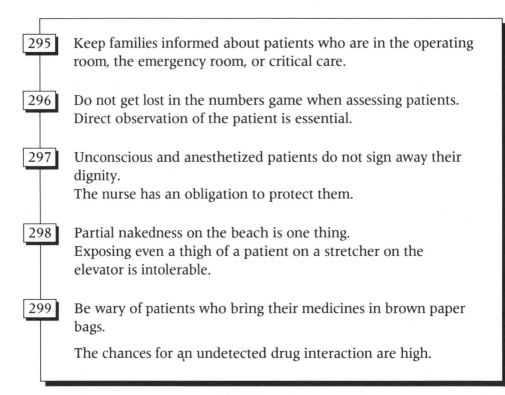

| 295 | Keep families informed about patients who are in the operating room, the emergency room, or critical care. |

| 296 | Do not get lost in the numbers game when assessing patients. Direct observation of the patient is essential. |

| 297 | Unconscious and anesthetized patients do not sign away their dignity. The nurse has an obligation to protect them. |

| 298 | Partial nakedness on the beach is one thing. Exposing even a thigh of a patient on a stretcher on the elevator is intolerable. |

| 299 | Be wary of patients who bring their medicines in brown paper bags. The chances for an undetected drug interaction are high. |

300   Patience gets short late in any shift.

301   Food should be:
    hot,
    recognizable,
    tasty, and
    within reach of the patient.

    Most of all, the meat should not be cold and greenish-brown.

302   The call bell is of no use if it is on the floor.

303   Do not become too familiar with a patient.
    You will lose your objectivity.
    It will prevent you from being an effective nurse.

304   Accept responsibility for each of your actions.

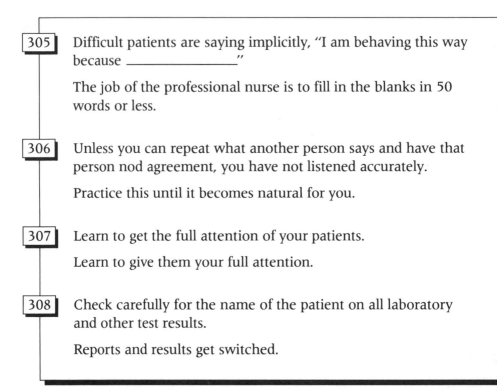

305 Difficult patients are saying implicitly, "I am behaving this way because _____"

The job of the professional nurse is to fill in the blanks in 50 words or less.

306 Unless you can repeat what another person says and have that person nod agreement, you have not listened accurately.

Practice this until it becomes natural for you.

307 Learn to get the full attention of your patients.

Learn to give them your full attention.

308 Check carefully for the name of the patient on all laboratory and other test results.

Reports and results get switched.

309   Learn to perform a detailed and thorough neurologic examination.

310   Some older people are fragile and decompensate easily. Be very gentle.

311   Much of what is called aging is simply disuse and inactivity.

Gently push older patients to stretch all their muscles daily and go for daily walks.

When you rest, you rust.

312   Learn to trust your feelings. They can tell you a lot about the emotional state of your patients.

If you feel depressed, the patient may be depressed.

If you feel confused, the patient may be confused or even demented.

313 Excellence in nursing is achievable.

Perfection is not.

Know the difference.

314 When talking with partially deaf patients, put your stethoscope in their ears and talk into the bell.

They will appreciate your thoughtfulness even if they still cannot hear.

315 Be wary of patients who bring their own pillows, especially if they are satin.

316 Always give patients the opportunity to tell you how they feel.

Only patients know how they feel.

No one else does.

317 Do not get angry with your patients if they do not improve according to your nursing care plan.

Do not get angry with your patients because of their life style.

Do not get angry with your patients.
If you do, get some help.

318 NEVER, NEVER connect the nasogastric tube to the tubing from the Foley catheter.

Flow in either direction is unfortunate.

319 If you find an unlabeled, filled syringe at the bedside, inject it into a sink,

never into a patient.

320 Never administer dry oxygen.
Be sure it is moistened.

321 There are several types of what is called noncompliance.

1. Patients who do not take prescribed drugs because they did not understand the instructions.

   Learn to communicate in the language of the patient.

2. Patients who do not take the recommended drugs because they do not trust the physician.

   Help them to build trust, if it is justified.

3. Patients who do not take prescribed drugs because they make them feel bad.

   Learn to hear these people.
   They are often correct.

322 If you cut off an arm band,
replace it immediately.

323 Be polite.

Ask patients how they want to be addressed.

Never call adults by their first name unless they insist on it.

324 THREE CARDINAL SINS OF A SURGICAL NURSE

Premedicating the wrong patient.

Prepping the wrong part of the body.

Sending the wrong patient for a procedure.

325 A response to a placebo does not prove the patient is faking the symptom.

After all, about 30% of people in drug trials with known diseases respond to the placebo.

326 All fecal impactions are preventable.

327 An unconscious patient's eyes are vulnerable.

Lubricate and patch them.

328 Never discuss patients on elevators.

All people on elevators are close relatives of your patients.

329 Anger overlies fear.
Do not respond to anger defensively.
Find out what the patient fears.

330 With patients who have extensive wounds with foul odors, try to make direct eye contact with the patient.

It will help you see the patient as a fellow human.

331 Learn to trust your intuition.

332 Many patients' image of a nurse is a white uniform and nursing cap.

Do not be offended if some people do not recognize you right away.

333 Florence Nightingale was the first nursing case manager.
Know as much about your patients as she knew about hers.

334 Some elderly patients like to stroke your arm.
It seems to calm them.

335 With loss of consciousness, hearing is the last sense to be lost and the first to return.

336 Music is healing.
Especially when the patient can choose it.

337 All elderly patients have already been your age.
You have not been their age.

Who knows more about life?

238 Never enter a patient's room without knocking or announcing yourself.

339 Never remove these two books from the patient's room:

The Holy Bible.
The telephone directory.

340 Keep a patient's teeth and mouth as clean as you want your own.

341 Learn when and when not to call a physician.

342 Always call the physician when:

There is a significant deterioration in the clinical state of the
patient.

The patient threatens to leave the hospital.

The wrong dose or drug has been given.

A laboratory test result is greatly abnormal or at a life-
threatening level.

The patient has a seizure.

The patient falls out of bed.

The patient refuses to accept treatments.

The patient or the family do not know what is going on.

The patient or family member become so angry that you are
unable to assuage it.

and . . .

Especially when a patient looks you in the eye and says he is
going to die before morning.

343 There is a time for action.

There is a time for no action.

344 There is only one way to learn the true art of nursing:

At the bedside with an experienced mentor as your guide.

345 Patients cannot read your mind.

Please explain in great detail what will happen with any procedure.

346 Read Florence Nightingale's *Notes on Nursing: What It Is and What It Is Not.**

---

* Nightingale F: Notes on Nursing: What It Is and What It Is Not. New York, Appleton Century Company, 1938.

347

There are times when scientific medicine has nothing more to offer a patient.

This is the unique time when nurses have everything to offer:

comfort,
compassion,
caring,
understanding, and
empathy.

If you would like to suggest a rule for the next edition, please photocopy this page as many times as needed and submit to the publisher. For information about ordering bulk quantities of the book for educational purposes, contact the publisher at 215-546-7293.

Nurses' Rules
c/o Hanley & Belfus, Inc.
210 South 13th Street
Philadelphia, PA 19107

Rule: _____

_____

_____

_____

_____

_____

From (name and address): _____

_____

_____